High Triglycerides Diet

A Beginner's 3-Week Step-by-Step Guide With Curated Recipes and a 7-Day Meal Plan

Copyright © 2020 Larry Jamesonn
All rights reserved. No portion of this book may be reproduced in any form without permission from the publisher, except as permitted by U.S. copyright law.

Disclaimer

By reading this disclaimer, you are accepting the terms of the disclaimer in full. If you disagree with this disclaimer, please do not read the guide. The content in this guide is provided for informational and educational purposes only.

This guide is not intended to be a substitute for the original work of this diet plan. At most, this guide is intended to be a beginner's supplement to the original work for this diet plan and never act as a direct substitute. This guide is an overview, review, and commentary on the facts of that diet plan.

All product names, diet plans, or names used in this guide are for identification purposes only and are the property of their respective owners. The use of these names does not imply endorsement. All other trademarks cited herein are the property of their respective owners.

None of the information in this guide should be accepted as independent medical or other professional advice.

The information in the guide has been compiled from various sources that are deemed reliable. It has been analyzed and summarized to the best of the Author's ability, knowledge, and belief. However, the Author cannot guarantee the accuracy and thus should not be held liable for any errors.

You acknowledge and agree that the Author of this guide will not be held liable for any damages, costs, expenses, resulting from the application of the information in this guide, whether directly or indirectly. You acknowledge and agree that you assume all risk and responsibility for any action you undertake in response to the information in this guide.

You acknowledge and agree that by continuing to read this guide, you will (where applicable, appropriate, or necessary) consult a qualified medical professional on this information. The information in this guide is not intended to be any sort of medical advice and should not be used instead of any medical advice by a licensed and qualified medical professional.

Always seek the advice of your physician or another qualified health provider with any issues or questions you might have regarding any sort of medical condition. Do not ever disregard any qualified professional medical advice or delay seeking that advice because of anything you have read in this guide.

Table of Contents

Introduction   6

Chapter 1: All About High Triglyceride Levels   9

Chapter 2: Consequences of High Triglyceride Levels   18

Chapter 3: How to Lower Triglyceride Levels   22

Chapter 4: Week 1 – Head start with the High Triglycerides Diet   25

Chapter 5: Week 2 – What Foods to Choose for Your Week's Meal   35

Chapter 6: Week 3 – Execute Everything Regularly   40

Sample Recipes for Inspiration   46

Conclusion   59

Introduction

Based on the gathered results from the National Health and Nutrition Examination Survey from 2001-2012, 25.1% of adult Americans aged 20 and older have increased triglyceride levels (>150 mg/dL) during 2009-2012. Although this was lower than the 33.3% prevalence in 2001-2004, it is still alarming given the current lifestyle of Americans which involves consumption of mostly processed and fast foods, and a sedentary lifestyle that contributes to increased prevalence of obesity. [1]

Increased triglyceride levels are said to be related to cardiovascular diseases such as heart attack, heart failure, and stroke. [2] And according to the Harvard Medical School, having high triglyceride levels may be an indication of a metabolic syndrome such as diabetes and pancreatitis.[3]

Because of the complications associated with high triglycerides, it is recommended that those with high triglyceride levels engage in beneficial lifestyles such as increasing physical activities, losing weight, quitting smoking, and having a balanced diet. [4] [5]

---

[1] https://www.cdc.gov/nchs/products/databriefs/db198.htm#:~:text=A%20greater%20percentage%20of%20men%20aged%2040%E2%80%9359%20(34.9%25),%25%20ofor%2060%20and%20over).

[2] Austin MA, Hokanson JE, Edwards KL. Hypertriglyceridemia as a cardiovascular risk factor. Am J Cardiol 81(4A):7B–12B. 1998.

[3] https://www.health.harvard.edu/heart-health/should-you-worry-about-high-triglycerides

However, it is difficult to monitor if you have high triglyceride levels because having this condition does not entail visible and characteristic symptoms. There are no recorded symptoms specific for having high triglycerides alone. [6] The only way to know if you have high triglycerides is through a blood test that will assess your lipid profile.

Now, you may have already started wondering about what triglycerides are exactly? And how does it affect your overall condition? These questions will be answered throughout this guide. But to give you a hint: it is a type of lipid that can be found in our bodies performing an array of functions.

In this guide, you are expected to learn more about the following:
- What are triglycerides?
- What are the functions of triglycerides in your body?
- What are considered normal levels of triglycerides?

---

[4] National Institutes of Health, National Heart, Lung, and Blood Institute. Third report of the National Cholesterol Education Program (NCEP) Expert Panel on Detection, Evaluation, and Treatment of High Blood Cholesterol in Adults (Adult treatment panel III): Final report. NIH publication no. 02–5215. 2002.

[5] Miller M, Stone NJ, Ballantyne C, Bittner V, Criqui MH, Ginsberg HN, et al. Triglycerides and cardiovascular disease: A scientific statement from the American Heart Association. Circulation 123(20):2292–333. 2011.

[6] https://www.nhlbi.nih.gov/health-topics/high-blood-triglycerides

- Why is it bad if your triglyceride levels are high?
- What can you do to manage to have high triglycerides?

Chapter 1: All About High Triglyceride Levels

What are Triglycerides

Triglycerides are a type of fat that can be found in the blood. [7] It came from the words: "tri" meaning three, and "glyceride", meaning glycerol, alcohol that serves as the backbone of different types of fats. Thus, this makes triglyceride a compound composed of three molecules of fatty acid together with a molecule of one alcohol glycerol. [8]

Triglycerides are the most common type of fat that can be found in our bodies since they come from foods that we commonly consume. These foods include oils, butter, and other fats from our diet. Also, when the body does not need the calories accumulated, they turn these calories into triglycerides and store them for later use. [9]

Although usually interchanged, triglycerides and cholesterol are different. Cholesterol, specifically the VLDL (very-low-density-lipoproteins), carries triglycerides in our blood. Hence, if you have a high VLDL cholesterol level, you are most likely to have a high triglyceride level, too. [10]

---

[7] https://www.mayoclinic.org/diseases-conditions/high-blood-cholesterol/in-depth/triglycerides/art-20048186
[8] https://www.medicinenet.com/triglycerides/definition.htm
[9] https://medlineplus.gov/triglycerides.html
[10] https://my.clevelandclinic.org/health/articles/17583-triglycerides--heart-health

This explains the occasion when testing for triglycerides level. The lipid profile which includes the different types of cholesterols is also made by the physician. This is because they are closely related, and they affect each other's quantities.

What do triglycerides do in our body?
Even though triglycerides are commonly associated with negative effects such as increased health risks, they still have a role they play in our bodies. These are the following: [11]

- **They provide energy to our bodies.** It was mentioned that triglycerides are calories that were turned into fat. And fat is a macronutrient that provides energy to the body. So, when we do not have available calories to use, these fats are broken down to become the energy we use to perform tasks.

- **They are the main storage of energy in the body.** As mentioned, calories are stored in the form of fat when not in use. These fats include triglycerides.

- **They protect and insulate the body.** Fats are great insulators because they are

---

[11]https://med.libretexts.org/Bookshelves/Nutrition/Book%3A_Intermediate_Nutrition_(Lindshield)/02%3A_Macronutrient_Structures/2.03%3A_Lipids/2.3E%3A_Triglycerides

hydrophobic, meaning they are water-fearing, thus, do not allow mixing with water. Also, there has been a study involving the relationship between the body mass index and being stabbed. The study found out that people with increased BMI are less likely to be severely injured than very thin patients. [12] This study implies that fat may protect our bodies from external force and injuries because they act as a "cushion."

- **They help in transporting and absorbing fat-soluble vitamins.** Vitamins are divided into two categories: water-soluble and fat-soluble. Each category needs water, and fat, respectively, to be used. Without these, they are useless. So, having fat in the body is essential to gain the benefits of fat-soluble vitamins we get from our food.

---

[12] Bloom MB, Ley EJ, Liou DZ, Tran T, Chung R, Melo N, Margulies DR. Impact of body mass index on injury in abdominal stab wounds: implications for management. J Surg Res. 2015 Jul;197(1):162-6. DOI: 10.1016/j.jss.2015.03.052. Epub 2015 Mar 26. PMID: 25891677.

Triglycerides Normal Levels

If they do well with the functions mentioned above, then why is it not good to have high triglyceride levels? This question will be answered in the next parts.

But let us first discuss the normal triglyceride levels to give you more ample background about triglycerides. The table below shows the different levels of triglycerides and their corresponding interpretations. [13]

Concentrations	Interpretation
<150 mg/dL	Normal
151-200 mg/dL	Borderline High
201-499 mg/dL	High
≥500 mg/dL	Very High

Studies have shown that having high triglyceride levels pose an increased risk of developing cardiovascular diseases such as stroke, heart failure, and heart attack. [14] It may also indicate the presence of diabetes and pancreatitis, which are metabolic syndromes. [15]

---

[13] https://my.clevelandclinic.org/health/articles/17583-triglycerides--heart-health

[14] Austin MA, Hokanson JE, Edwards KL. Hypertriglyceridemia as a cardiovascular risk factor. Am J Cardiol 81(4A):7B–12B. 1998.

[15] https://www.health.harvard.edu/heart-health/should-you-worry-about-high-triglycerides

How to know if your triglycerides are high

As mentioned, you cannot suspect if you have high triglycerides because it does not show symptoms. What you can do is schedule a triglyceride level test or the triacylglycerol test regularly to constantly determine the current number of triglycerides in your blood.

The triacylglycerol test helps in estimating the LDL (low-density lipoprotein) cholesterol or the "bad cholesterol" in your blood which carries your triglycerides around the body. The test may also tell if you are at risk of having atherosclerosis, pancreatitis, or heart disease.

This test is ideally taken every five years. In this test, you will find out the HDL, LDL, cholesterol, and triglyceride concentrations in your body—or your lipid profile. However, if you have pre-existing diabetes, you are required to do the test more frequently because triglyceride levels will increase if your blood glucose levels are not maintained properly.

Taking the test to have its conditions since triglycerides are sensitive to food and other medications. The following are what you need to do before the test: [16]

---

[16] https://www.healthline.com/health/triglyceride-level#procedure

- **Do fast.** It is recommended to fast for 9-14 hours before the test. This means that water is the only thing you can take. You may also refer to the doctor's instructions regarding the fasting period. Also, avoiding alcohol for 24 hours before the test is highly recommended. Tip: Schedule your test in the morning so you are already fasting while you are sleeping.

- **Inform the doctor about your medications.** Medicine such as Vitamin C, estrogens, birth control pills, retinoids, some antipsychotics, statins, etc. affects the results of the test. So, tell your doctor about your medications so he/she will guide you on what medications are fine and what are not.

What to expect during the triglyceride test

The triglyceride test uses your blood sample. Then, it is brought to the medical laboratory for analysis. You do not need to worry because the test is performed by a healthcare professional and they generally follow the following steps in getting your blood sample:
1. The healthcare professional will clean first the area where they will get the blood with an antiseptic. To easily locate and fill your veins with blood, an elastic band will be wrapped around your arm.

2. You will be injected with a needle connected with a tube wherein your blood is collected.
3. When the tube is already full, they will remove the elastic band first, and then the needle. To stop bleeding, they will press a gauze or cotton ball against the puncture.

Since blood is collected from your body, you may feel mild discomfort or pain. In some cases, having your blood tested may cause fainting, lightheadedness, excessive bleeding, infection, or the buildup of blood under the skin called a hematoma.

Testing glycerides may also be made by purchasing a portable machine that analyzes the lipid profile of a small amount of blood (blood from a finger prick). These machines may cost around $70 to $150 depending on the brand and are usually seen during medical and health fairs.

What does it mean if you have high triglycerides?
Mentioned in the table above are the ranges which determine a certain interpretation of your triglyceride levels. If you have increased levels, your condition is called hypertriglyceridemia, which means "condition of having more triglycerides".

If you have 1,000 mg/dL or greater, you are at risk of developing pancreatitis, the inflammation of the pancreas. You should inform your doctor about this to help you reverse the effects immediately.

If your triglycerides are high, your bad cholesterol is also high. So, proper treatment and diagnosis from the doctor are recommended.

Causes of high triglycerides
Having high triglycerides may come from various sources. Some of them may be due to an unhealthy lifestyle or pre-existing medical conditions. Listed below are lifestyle habits that may have contributed to your elevated triglyceride levels:
- Obesity or being overweight
- Alcohol consumption
- Binge drinking
- Low-protein diet
- High-carbohydrate diet
- Smoking
- Inactivity

While below are medical conditions that may have influenced your increased triglyceride levels. These are:
- Diabetes
- Unmaintained blood sugar levels
- Genetics
- Cirrhosis
- Hyperthyroidism
- Hyperlipidemia

- Pancreatitis
- Kidney disease

Also, they may be caused by your current medications such as[17]

- Birth control oils
- Retinoids
- Diuretics
- Steroids
- A few immunosuppressants
- Some HIV prescription medication
- Beta-blockers

Diagnosis and Treatment

Hypertriglyceridemia is the clinical term for having elevated levels of triglycerides. This condition is usually treated through lifestyle changes or medications.

But one of the most effective and widely used treatments to control your triglyceride levels is a lifestyle change. This involves increased physical activities and more mindful eating.

---

[17] https://www.mayoclinic.org/diseases-conditions/high-blood-cholesterol/in-depth/triglycerides/art-20048186#:~:text=Your%20doctor%20will%20usually%20check,for%20an%20accurate%20triglyceride%20measurement.

Chapter 2: Consequences of High Triglyceride Levels

Consequences of having high triglyceride levels

It is important to continuously check your triglycerides level because having too little or too much is crucial. Also, it has no symptoms so you will have to see for yourself or experience the consequences later.

Having high triglycerides is associated with a wide array of diseases that does not only compromise your health but your overall wellbeing as well. To give you some, here is a list of diseases related to having high triglycerides. [18] [19]

- **Coronary artery disease.** Triglycerides are now thought to be a risk factor for various cardiovascular diseases such as coronary artery disease. When triglyceride levels are elevated, the metabolism of cholesterol is also altered, thus, increasing the risk of developing heart diseases.[20] Also, since triglycerides are fat, they tend to cause plaque buildup along the walls of the arteries of the heart, in charge of supplying blood to the

---

[18] https://emedicine.medscape.com/article/126568-overview

[19] https://www.mayoclinic.org/diseases-conditions/high-blood-cholesterol/in-depth/triglycerides/art-20048186#:~:text=High%20triglycerides%20may%20contribute%20to,of%20the%20pancreas%20(pancreatitis).

[20] McBride P. Triglycerides and risk for coronary artery disease. Curr Atheroscler Rep. 2008 Oct;10(5):386-90. DOI: 10.1007/s11883-008-0060-9. PMID: 18706279.

other parts of the body, causing high blood pressure and sometimes, heart attack. [21]

- **Hyperlipoproteinemia.** This is a metabolic disorder wherein there are abnormally increased levels of lipoproteins such as cholesterols. It is associated with high triglyceride levels because the LDL or "bad cholesterol" is the triglyceride carrier. So, if one of them is at high concentrations, the other is most likely to have elevated levels, too.

- **Type 2 diabetes or prediabetes.** Studies have shown a link between high triglyceride levels and insulin resistance. [22] Insulin is a hormone released by the pancreas to control blood sugar levels. [23] So, if you are insulin resistant, your cells cannot respond well to insulin's effects. Thus, your blood sugar levels are not changing as desired. [24]

- **Pancreatitis.** About insulin resistance, it is considered fine if your cells are not responding well to the insulin if the pancreas

---

[21] https://www.cdc.gov/heartdisease/coronary_ad.htm#:~:text=Coronary%20Artery%20Disease%20(CAD),arteries%20to%20narrow%20over%20time.
[22] https://www.verywellhealth.com/what-causes-high-triglycerides-in-diabetes-1087722#citation-3
[23] https://www.endocrineweb.com/conditions/type-1-diabetes/what-insulin
[24] https://www.niddk.nih.gov/health-information/diabetes/overview/what-is-diabetes/prediabetes-insulin-resistance#:~:text=Insulin%20resistance%20is%20when%20cells,help%20glucose%20enter%20your%20cells.

is still healthy and working. But, in the case of pancreatitis, the pancreas is inflamed, thus, making its work compromised.

- **Hypothyroidism.** It is a condition when the thyroid gland fails to make enough thyroid hormones that are in charge of maintaining metabolic health. [25] [26] This condition is associated with high triglycerides because it causes elevated LDL cholesterol levels, which then carry the triglycerides.

- **Genetics.** Some genes poorly break down triglycerides, thus, failing to control these levels in the body. One of the conditions involving genetics is familial hypertriglyceridemia that is passed from one generation to another. [27]

- **Atherosclerosis.** Just like coronary artery disease, atherosclerosis is also caused by the accumulation of fatty deposits in the arteries. These deposits are made up of cholesterol and triglycerides. [28]

---

[25] https://www.yourhormones.info/glands/thyroid-gland/#:~:text=The%20thyroid%20gland%20produces%20hormones,of%20iodine%20from%20the%20diet.

[26] https://www.thyroid.org/hypothyroidism/#:~:text=Hypothyroidism%20is%20an%20underactive%20thyroid,thyroid%20hormone%20in%20the%20blood.

[27] https://www.webmd.com/cholesterol-management/familial-hypertriglyceridemia#:~:text=Some%20people%20have%20high%20triglycerides%20and%20aren't%20physically%20active.

[28] https://www.health.harvard.edu/heart-health/know-your-triglycerides-heres-why#:~:text=The%20level%20of%20triglycerides%20in,your%20risk%20for%20heart%20disease.&text=Low%2Ddensity%20lipoprotein%20(LDL),to%20heart%20attacks%20and%20strokes.

Are there good benefits to having high triglyceride levels?

Triglycerides are complex compounds of fats. And they serve different purposes in our bodies. They act as:
- Reserved energy
- Protection
- Insulation
- Absorbers of fat-soluble vitamins
- Transporters

But it is safe to say that everything too little or too high is not good. Even the vitamins and minerals can be toxic if excessive. So, in the case of triglycerides, it is recommended to maintain it at a normal level to benefit from the said purposes, instead of experiencing the consequences.

Chapter 3: How to Lower Triglyceride Levels

By this time, you may have already considered taking the triglyceride test. So, what will you do if you have elevated levels of triglycerides?

Studies generally suggest the following: [29]

- **Engage in a more active lifestyle.** One of the causes of high triglyceride levels is having excess energy that is not burned. Through a more active lifestyle, excess calories are burned instead of just being stored in the body.

- **Start a healthier diet.** If you eat excess calories and cannot burn them, the excess calories will just be stored as fat. So, being a mindful eater where you know your limits on how much food you can eat is essential to control the high triglyceride level concentrations in your body.

- **Some medications.** In some cases where lifestyle change is enough or, some organs such as the pancreas are not working properly, medications are recommended by the physicians. Examples

---

[29] https://www.mayoclinic.org/diseases-conditions/high-blood-cholesterol/in-depth/triglycerides/art-20048186#:~:text=High%20triglycerides%20may%20contribute%20to,of%20the%20pancreas%20(pancreatitis).

of these medications are statins, niacin, fibrates, and even fish oil.

In this guide, we will focus on how to control your elevated triglycerides level through a low-triglyceride diet.

What to eat and what not to eat in this diet?

Fats are essential macronutrients that we need to consume in our daily lives because they provide us with our daily energy needs. It is a misconception that fats are generally bad because it is almost always associated with lifestyle and non-communicable diseases such as hypertension, cardiovascular diseases, and diabetes. [30]

But in reality, fats are needed by the body to perform their different functions. In actuality, up to 30% of your caloric intake should come from fat. [31] So, the principle of this diet is not to exclude and neglect all of your fats. The key to doing this diet is choosing your foods wisely (like choosing between saturated and unsaturated fat).

---

[30] https://www.hsph.harvard.edu/nutritionsource/what-should-you-eat/fats-and-cholesterol/types-of-fat/

[31] https://wa.kaiserpermanente.org/healthAndWellness/?item=%2Fcommon%2FhealthAndWellness%2Fconditions%2Fdiabetes%2FfoodBalancing.html#:~:text=In%20a%20healthy%20diet%2C%20about%2030%20percent%20of%20total%20daily,percent%20of%20fat%20into%20glucose.

So, you can eat anything you want as long as it is a healthier choice. But since you are managing your high triglycerides, you cannot be too lax with your intake. It is still important to watch out for the components of your food. In the succeeding chapters, you will be given tips on how to choose your foods wisely, how to cook and choose your meals, and how to sustain your current lifestyle.

Chapter 4: Week 1 – Head start with the High Triglycerides Diet

To help you head start your first week of the triglyceride-controlled diet, the following are just some tips when choosing food items to consume:

- **Choose unsaturated fats over saturated and trans-fat.**[32]
  Different types of fat exist in different forms. Unsaturated fats are fats that are liquid at room temperature. They are the "healthy" fats because they help ease inflammations, soothe heart rhythms, and improve blood cholesterol concentrations. Unsaturated fats mainly come from plants.

  On the other hand, we have saturated fats which are solid at room temperature, and examples are fat from cheese, beef, ice cream, palm oil, and coconut oil. Too much of this type of fat may also be a precursor to diabetes. [33]

  Lastly, we have trans fats which are processed vegetable oils through hydrogenation. This is the type of fat you would want to avoid the most because it contributes to insulin resistance, starts

---

[32] https://www.hsph.harvard.edu/nutritionsource/what-should-you-eat/fats-and-cholesterol/types-of-fat/

[33] Riserus, U., W.C. Willett, and F.B. Hu, Dietary fats and prevention of type 2 diabetes. *Prog Lipid Res*, 2009. 48(1): p. 44-51.

inflammation, lowers good cholesterol, and raises bad cholesterol. Examples of trans fat are fried foods in lard, margarine, pizza, and even baked goods.

Also, if you use saturated fats in cooking multiple times, these become trans fat and are carcinogenic or cancerous.
Fish oils are also ideal for your fat intake as they contain omega-3 fatty acids that have long been recommended because it is good for the heart.

- **Consume more fruits, vegetables, and low-fat products.** [34]
Fruits and vegetables are generally healthier options when it comes to food. They contain nutrients such as vitamins and minerals that help regulate body functions.

In the triglyceride diet, it is recommended to consume more of these food items because they also have fiber which helps in eliminating bad cholesterol. They also help in metabolism and other digestive functions.

Fruits and vegetables also contain fewer calories than processed and fast foods. So, you can eat more of these, but you only

---

[34] https://www.everydayhealth.com/heart-health/diet-tips-to-reduce-high-triglycerides.aspx

consume a few calories. The fiber also helps you feel satiated so that you do not feel like you are eating less.

As per other products such as milk, and other dairy products, some options are low-fat or even nonfat. Choosing these over whole-fat products makes a huge difference in helping you control your triglyceride levels.

- **Drink alcohol in moderation.**
Did you know that if you do not burn the alcoholic calories for 24 hours, they are turned into fat on your belly? This is where the beer belly term came from.

  So, it will not hurt if you will slow down on your alcohol intake if you do not have many physical activities that you can execute.

  Also, alcohol digestion takes place in your liver, thus, the more alcohol you consume, the more work it gives to your liver.

- **Opt for low-fat protein**
Opting for low-fat meat such as fish, beans, chicken, soy, and lean meats will help you control your triglyceride levels. Fat, whether visible or not visible, are still fats contained in the meat.

Also, the fat in animal products is usually saturated fats that may contribute to clogging veins and vessels if taken excessively.

Exploring other cooking methods that do not make use of oil such as boiling, baking, or simmering is also ideal when serving proteins. This makes sure that you are not getting more fat than you should.

- **Avoid added sugars** [35]
Sweets may be a delight to your taste buds, but your liver may convert the excess sugar you consume into triglycerides. Sugars do not necessarily exist as the granulated ones you use in your coffee. You may be shocked to know where you get these added sugars from. Examples are candy, soda, baked goods, breakfast cereals, fruit juices, ice cream, and yogurt.

   Although fruits also contain sugars, they are healthier because they are natural and not processed compared to the sugars in the examples above.

For you to have the first week easy, below is a sample meal plan you can use for the first week.

---

[35] https://www.medicinenet.com/lower_triglycerides_pictures_slideshow/article.htm

Monday	**Breakfast** Rice bran flakes with bananas and skimmed milk **AM Snack** Low-fat or Non-fat yogurt with Choice Berries **Lunch** Whole-Wheat Pita Sandwich with Grilled Turkey and String Cheese **PM Snack** Mixed Fruits Salad **Dinner** Broiled Cod with tomatoes and cheese Couscous with Steamed Broccoli Sprouts
Tuesday	**Breakfast** Berries Low-fat Smoothie Organic Hard-boiled Eggs **AM Snack** Unsalted and unbuttered

	popcorn **Lunch** Vegan Soup with Vegan Burger Steak in Whole-Wheat Sandwich Toast Muffins **PM Snack** Apple and Berries **Dinner** Grilled Chicken Breast Fillet in Rosemary and Thyme Baked Sweet Potato
Wednesday	**Breakfast** High-protein oats in Almond Milk and Honey Tops **AM Snack** Yogurt with nuts and Berries **Lunch** Grilled Chicken California Salad **PM Snack** Spinach and Watercress Salad

	Dinner Steamed Shrimp Salad with Spinach and Greek Yogurt Dressing
Thursday	**Breakfast** English Muffins and Sliced Apples **AM Snack** Greek Yogurt **Lunch** Tomato Soup with Lean Ground Beef and Fresh Lettuce Hummus and Raw Vegetables Brown Rice **PM Snack** Mixed Fruit Salads **Dinner** Baked Salmon with Coleslaw and Quinoa Grains
Friday	**Breakfast**

	Spinach and Tomato Omelet **AM Snack** Low-fat or Non-fat yogurt with Choice Berries **Lunch** Low-fat Cheese Quesadilla with Mixed Vegetables, Salsa, and Guacamole **PM Snack** Mixed Fruits Salad **Dinner** Roasted Pork Loin Mashed Squash and Leafy Greens
Saturday	**Breakfast** Whole-Wheat Fresh Waffle Sandwich with Sliced Bananas and Peanut Butter **AM Snack** Fresh fruit juice **Lunch** Pescatarian Tacos with Tuna

	PM Snack Unsalted whole-grain crackers **Dinner** Jambalaya with Brown Rice, Turkey, and Mixed Beans
Sunday	**Breakfast** Toasted Cheese and Spinach on English Muffin **AM Snack** Sliced Fruits **Lunch** Black Beans Salad with Mandarin and Vinaigrette Dressing **PM Snack** Mixed Fruits **Dinner** Broiled Beef Flank with Baked Zucchini and Sweet Potato Wedges

Chapter 5: Week 2 – What Foods to Choose for Your Week's Meal

Now that you are on your second week of the diet. It is expected that you may have already picked up some tips on how to choose foods you will eat. So, this week, take your knowledge to the test and see if the meal plan below matches your "dream" meal plan.

Monday	**Breakfast** Egg Whites on Whole Wheat Bread with Peanut Butter Spread Sliced Apple Brewed Coffee **AM Snack** Fruits with Low-fat string cheese Unsalted Popcorn and without butter **Lunch** Chicken Salad with Vinaigrette Dressing, Whole Grain Crackers

	Sugar-free Lemonade **PM Snack** Low-fat or Non-fat yogurt with Choice Berries **Dinner** Baked salmon with almonds Brown rice and Stir-fry Vegetables
Tuesday	**Breakfast** Low-cholesterol Swiss Asparagus Omelet **AM Snack** Mixed Fruits Salad **Lunch** Roast Veggies **PM Snack** Unsalted and unbuttered popcorn **Dinner** Seafood Stew
Wednesday	**Breakfast** Breakfast Smoothie

	AM Snack Apple and Berries **Lunch** Grenade Salad **PM Snack** Yogurt with nuts and Berries **Dinner** Grilled Lamb with roast veggies
Thursday	**Breakfast** Spinach and Tomato Omelet **AM Snack** Spinach and Watercress Salad **Lunch** Broiled lean pork with tamarind soup Brown Rice **PM Snack** Mixed Fruit Salads **Dinner** Chicken Pad Thai

Friday	**Breakfast** Egg Whites on Whole Wheat Bread with Peanut Butter Spread **AM Snack** Mixed Fruits Salad **Lunch** Tomato Clams **PM Snack** Low-fat or Non-fat yogurt with Choice Berries **Dinner** Baked Flounder
Saturday	**Breakfast** Peanut butter and Banana Milkshake **AM Snack** Unsalted whole-grain crackers **Lunch** Salmon and Asparagus **PM Snack** Fresh fruit juice

	Dinner Mixed Vegetable Roast with Lemon Zest
Sunday	**Breakfast** Spinach and Watercress Salad **AM Snack** Mixed Fruits **Lunch** Arugula Mushroom Salad **PM Snack** Sliced Fruits **Dinner** Egg rolls and sauce

Is this how you wanted to plan your meals? If it is, then you are ready to continue this diet! If not, it is okay. You are just starting to do this diet, and no pressure is put on you. Just make sure to review the tips that you have learned in the first week and apply them as you continue along with your diet.

Chapter 6: Week 3 — Execute Everything Regularly

Now, you have already seen what your weekly meal would look like with this diet. Just remember that this diet will not work if it is used alone. It is best to remember these tips to ensure that you can continue doing this diet and start to take control of your triglyceride levels:

- Do exercise regularly
- Make the diet a habit
- Do not starve yourself
- Do not binge eat
- Be a mindful eater

As a bonus, here is another week's plan before you do it all by yourself. We also collected some of the recipes of the dishes in the meal plan for you to enjoy!

Monday	**Breakfast** Oatmeal with mixed berries, fruit nuts, and cocoa nibs **AM Snack** Sliced Peaches and Apple in Dark Chocolate **Lunch** Roast Chicken Breast in Lettuce Wraps with Avocado

	and Tomatoes **PM Snack** Vegetable Salad with Hard-boiled Eggs **Dinner** Baked Chicken and Broccoli Sticks with Brown Rice
Tuesday	**Breakfast** Whole-Grain Muffins with Grapes and Peanut Butter **AM Snack** Fresh Mixed Berries **Lunch** Avocado Pasta with Celery, Bell Pepper, and Baby Carrots **PM Snack** Greek Yogurt with Quinoa Grains **Dinner** Shrimp Fajitas in Whole-Wheat Pita
Wednesda	**Breakfast**

y	Cooked Oats with Greek Yogurt and Mixed Berries

AM Snack
Unsalted Popcorn and Fresh Cheese

Lunch
Broiled lean pork with tamarind soup

Brown Rice

PM Snack
Yogurt with nuts and Berries

Dinner
Cheesy Broccoli and Quinoa Casserole

Santa Fe Chicken Salad |
| Thursday | **Breakfast**
Spinach and Tomato Omelet

AM Snack
Tiny Celery Sticks and Hummus

Lunch |

	Turkey-and-Quinoa-Stuffed Bell Peppers **PM Snack** Mixed Fruit Salads **Dinner** Shrimp Pad Thai
Friday	**Breakfast** Peanut butter and Banana Milkshake **AM Snack** Fresh fruit juice **Lunch** Tomato Clams **PM Snack** Unsalted whole-grain crackers **Dinner** Baked Flounder
Saturday	**Breakfast** Egg Whites on Whole Wheat Bread with Peanut Butter Spread

	AM Snack Low-fat or Non-fat yogurt with Choice Berries **Lunch** Vegetarian Quesadillas **PM Snack** Fresh fruit juice **Dinner** Vegetarian Burger Patties in Whole-Wheat Toast
Sunday	**Breakfast** Greek Yogurt with Sliced Apples, Bananas, Blueberries, Strawberries, and Granola **AM Snack** Spinach and Watercress Salad **Lunch** Chicken Tortilla Wraps with Tomatoes and Guacamole **PM Snack** Mixed Fruits **Dinner** Basil and Strawberry Salad

Sample Recipes for Inspiration

__Roasted Veggies__

Ingredients:
- 1/2 lb. turnips
- 1/2 lb. carrots
- 1/2 lb. parsnips
- 2 shallots, peeled
- 1/4 tsp. ground black pepper
- 1 tbsps. extra-virgin olive oil
- 6 cloves garlic
- 3/4 tsp. kosher salt
- 2 tbsp. fresh rosemary needles

Instructions:
1. First, cut vegetables into bite-sized pieces.
2. Set the oven to 400°F.
3. Mix all the ingredients in a baking dish.
4. Roast the vegetables for 25 minutes until brown and tender.
5. Toss and roast again for 20- 25 minutes.
6. Serve and enjoy while hot.

Grilled Lamb

Ingredients:
- 1-1/2 lb. baby spinach leaves
- 3 tbsp. dried oregano, chopped
- 1/4 cup lemon juice
- 1/4 cup olive oil
- 2 tbsp. ground cumin
- 1 tsp. crushed red pepper
- 1 tbsp. coarse sea salt
- 1 tbsp. squeezed juice from an orange
- 3 cloves garlic
- 2 yellow onions, chopped
- cooking spray

Instructions:
1. In a 2-gallon zip bag, put the lamb together with the lemon juice, oregano, cumin, and salt.
2. Close the bag and refrigerate overnight
3. Puree onions, garlic, some orange juice, and olive oil in a blender.
4. Transfer to a small bowl with a cover.
5. Chill overnight.
6. Mix sea salt, red pepper, and cumin in a small bowl
7. Remove refrigerated lamb and let it sit for 30 minutes.
8. Preheat the grill to medium.
9. Place lamb on the grill and coat with some cooking spray or oil.

10. Grill lamb for one and a half hours over medium heat.
11. Remove lamb from the grill.
12. Serve hot.

☐

Spinach and Watercress Salad

Ingredients:
- 1 cup watercress, washed with stems removed
- 3 cups baby spinach, washed with stems removed
- 1 medium sliced avocado
- 1/4 cup avocado oil
- 1/8 cup lemon juice
- a pinch of salt

Instructions:
1. Pat dry the spinach and watercress. Remove the stem and separate the leaves.
2. On a large serving plate, combine the leaves of the watercress and the spinach.
3. Cut the avocado in half then remove the pit. Peel the skin off from each side.
4. Slice the avocados into thin strips. Set aside.
5. Prepare the dressing by combining avocado oil and lemon juice.
6. Arrange the avocado strips on top of the watercress and spinach.
7. Season with salt and pepper.
8. Drizzle with the dressing before serving.

Mixed Vegetable Roast and Lemon Zest

Ingredients:
- 1-1/2 cups broccoli florets
- 1-1/2 cups cauliflower florets
- 3/4 cup red bell pepper, diced
- 3/4 cup zucchini, diced
- 2 thinly sliced cloves of garlic
- 2 tsp. lemon zest
- 1 tbsp. olive oil
- A pinch of salt
- 1 tsp. dried and crushed oregano

Instructions:
1. Preheat the oven at 425°F for 25 minutes.
2. Combine garlic and florets of broccoli and cauliflower in a baking pan.
3. Drizzle oil evenly over the vegetables. Season with salt and oregano.
4. Stir the vegetables to coat them evenly.
5. Place the pan inside the oven and roast for 10 minutes.
6. Add zucchini and bell pepper to the mix. Toss to combine.
7. Continue roasting for 10 to 15 minutes more until the vegetables turn light brown.
8. Drizzle lemon zest over vegetables and toss.
9. Serve and enjoy.

Salmon and Asparagus

Ingredients:
- 2 salmon fillets
- 14 ounces young potatoes
- 8 asparagus spears, trimmed and halved
- 2 handfuls cherry tomatoes
- 1 handful basil leaves
- 2 tbsp. extra-virgin olive oil
- 1 tbsp. balsamic vinegar

Instructions:
1. Heat oven to 428°F.
2. Arrange potatoes into a baking dish.
3. Drizzle potatoes with extra-virgin olive oil.
4. Roast potatoes until they have turned golden brown.
5. Place asparagus into the baking dish together with the potatoes.
6. Roast in the oven for 15 minutes.
7. Arrange cherry tomatoes and salmon among the vegetables.
8. Drizzle with balsamic vinegar and the remaining olive oil.
9. Roast until the salmon is cooked.
10. Throw in basil leaves before transferring everything to a serving dish.
11. Serve while hot.

Arugula and Mushroom Salad

Ingredients:
- 5 oz. arugula washed
- 1 lb. fresh mushrooms
- 1/4 teaspoon shoyu
- 1/2 red onion
- 1 tbsp. olive oil
- 1 tbsp. mirin

To make tofu cheese:
- 1/8 cup umeboshi vinegar
- 1/2 firm tofu

Instructions:
1. In a bowl, add the rinsed tofu. Crumble and pour in vinegar.
2. In a separate bowl add shoyu, red onions, salt, olive oil, and mirin. Mix to combine.
3. Add in the arugula and toss to combine with the dressing.
4. Serve and enjoy.

Grenade Salad

Ingredients:
- 4 cups arugula
- 1 large avocado
- 1/2 cup sliced fennel
- 1/2 cup sliced Anjou pears
- 1/4 cup pomegranate seeds

Instructions:
1. Mix all the ingredients except for the pomegranate seeds.
2. After mixing well, add the seeds. Mix again.
3. Serve with any type of desired dressing.

Seafood Stew

Ingredients:
- 2 tsp. extra-virgin olive oil
- 1 cut bulb fennel
- 2 stalks celery, chopped
- 2 cups white wine
- 1 tbsp. chopped thyme
- 1 cup chopped shallots
- 6 ounces shrimp
- 6 ounces of sea scallops
- 1/4 tsp. salt
- 1 cup chopped parsley
- 6 oz. Arctic char
- 2-1/2 cups of water

Instructions:
1. Heat a frying pan on the lowest setting. Add a small amount of oil.
2. Cook the celery, shallots, and fennel for approximately 6 minutes.
3. Pour in the wine, water, and thyme into the frying pan.
4. Wait for 10 minutes and allow it to cook.
5. Once much of the water has evaporated, add in the remaining ingredients, and wait for 2 minutes before removing from the stove.
6. Serve and enjoy immediately.

Tomato Clams

Ingredients:
- Canola oil cooking spray
- 1 onion, sliced
- 1 tsp. minced garlic, or to taste
- 1/2 tsp salt
- 3 pounds of clams, in shell, thoroughly scrubbed
- 1 tsp red pepper flakes
- 1 cup white wine
- 1/2 lb. whole-grain linguine, cooked according to package directions
- 1/2 cup flat-leaf parsley, chopped
- 4 cups cherry tomatoes, halved

Instructions:
1. Heat a large pot with a lid over low heat.
2. Spray with vegetable oil cooking spray and add the onion, garlic, and salt. Cook for 3 minutes, stirring constantly.
3. Add the clams, red pepper flakes, and wine
4. Cover and simmer until the clams open, approximately 7 minutes. Discard those clams that do not open.
5. Add the pasta, parsley, and tomatoes. Cover and let simmer for an additional 3 minutes. Stir and serve immediately.

Baked Flounder

Ingredients:
- 1 lb. flounder, filleted
- 1/4 tsp. salt
- 1 cup halved red grapes
- 1 tbsp. extra-virgin olive oil
- 2 tbsp. parsley, chopped finely
- 1 tbsp. lemon juice
- 1 cup almonds, chopped and toasted
- freshly ground black pepper, to taste

Instructions:
1. Preheat the oven to 375°F.
2. Place fish on a sheet tray. Season with olive oil, salt, and pepper.
3. Combine the almonds, grapes, lemon juice, parsley, 1-1/2 tsp. of olive oil, 1/8 tsp of salt, and black pepper in a bowl.
4. Bake the fish for about 3 minutes.
5. Flip the fish and return to the oven.
6. Bake for another 3 minutes, or until the fish is starting to flake, while the center is still translucent. Don't overcook.
7. Serve immediately, topped with the grape mixture.

Low-Cholesterol Swiss Asparagus Omelet

Ingredients:
- cooking spray
- 5 pieces of trimmed and cooked asparagus spears
- 3/4 cup of Egg Beaters Liquid Egg Whites
- 1 slice of halved Swiss cheese
- 1/8 teaspoon of ground black pepper

Instructions:
1. Spray small amounts of cooking spray in a nonstick skillet.
2. Place it over medium heat.
3. Add the Egg Beaters and cook for 2 minutes.
4. Lift the edges to cook the other side of the egg.
5. Cook for 3more minutes.
6. Top the half of the omelet with pepper, feta cheese, and asparagus.
7. Fold the other half of the omelet over the filling.
8. Slide to plate to serve.

Vegan Pesto

Ingredients:
- 1/3 cup olive oil (or other high-quality and flavorful oil)
- 1-1/2 cups basil, fresh
- 5 cloves garlic
- 1 cup pine nuts
- 1/3 cup nutritional yeast
- 3/4 teaspoon salt
- 1/2 teaspoon black pepper

Instructions:
1. In a food processor, add in all the ingredients.
2. Start processing until the nuts are ground.
3. Add more salt and pepper to taste.

Conclusion

Thank you again for getting this guide.

If you found this guide helpful, please take the time to share your thoughts and post a review. It'd be greatly appreciated!

Thank you and good luck!

Made in the USA
Monee, IL
01 April 2022